Mirror, Mirror on the Wall
Breaking the "I Feel Fat" Spell

Andrea Wachter, LMFT
and Marsea Marcus, LMFT

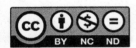 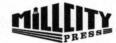
Cover Design by Michelle Fairbanks/Fresh Design
Cover and Interior Illustrations by Jennifer Kalis
Edited by Amanda Gawthorpe

ISBN 978-1-63505-301-2
Library of Congress Control Number: 2016908786

Table of Contents

For Parents, Counselors, and Other Concerned Adults

We have all had a massive hypnotic spell cast upon us, both children and adults alike. We are bombarded every single day with repetitive messages that tell us if we improve our bodies, we will find peace, happiness, and love. We are surrounded by people who worry about their weight and fret about food. The word "fat" has practically become a curse word in our image-obsessed culture when, in actuality, fat is something all bodies have in different places and amounts, at different times in our lives. Adult paranoia about fat has left many kids confused, fearing that any fat on their precious bodies means something bad about who they are. Some kids (and even some adults) think that eating fat should be completely avoided, rather than understanding that fat is an essential nutrient, necessary for providing energy, absorbing vitamins, insulating our bodies, and helping us feel satiated.

The demonization of fat has had far-reaching negative consequences, and as a result, body dissatisfaction and eating disorders have reached epidemic proportions. We have been brainwashed to believe that flat stomachs are somehow better than fleshy stomachs, that smaller clothing sizes are superior to larger ones, that weight loss equals success, and that fat people are intrinsically weak and unlovable. As a culture, we have succumbed to false ideas such as these, as if they were facts. Some of us are more susceptible to this brainwashing than others. Children certainly are. But the good news is that because they are young, their brains are more malleable, and they haven't been hypnotized as long as some adults have. Therefore, it's easier for kids to remember who they were before they got struck by the "I Feel Fat" Spell. It's also a lot easier to heal body image issues in the early stages, before they become embedded or morph into full-blown eating disorders. So early prevention is key!

While it is a tragedy that there is a need for a book such as this, it has become a reality that there is such a need. Whether you are a parent, a counselor, or another concerned adult, if you have, work with, or know a young child who suffers from a painful body image, the exercises in this book can help you help them.

Who This Book is For:

This book is designed for kids (12 and under) who have been struck by the "I Feel Fat" Spell. This spell can strike kids of any size, so how do you know if a child is caught in the spell? Maybe you hear them complain about the size or shape of their body. Perhaps they frequently compare themselves unfavorably to their friends. They tend to feel extremely uncomfortable, self-conscious, and anxious about their appearance. They often try to soothe their anxiety with behaviors such as restricting their food intake, overeating, over-exercising, limiting what they will wear, or refusing to do activities they once enjoyed. You may have noticed significant weight changes, or perhaps their physician has expressed concern. And though you may have tried to help them feel better about themselves, they continue to dislike, or even despise, their bodies. This book is for them.

We have also discovered that many adults are finding this book to be extremely helpful, if not life-changing. Some have told us that it appealed to the kid inside of them, while others found that the simplicity of the language helped them better understand the difficult concepts. We are thrilled that people of all ages are using this book to break the "I Feel Fat" Spell.

How to Use This Book:

Most children's books are read in one sitting, but it is our hope that with this book you will focus on one chapter at a time. Each chapter gives kids (and you) a lot to think about. We hope you and your child will take the time to discuss the lessons and start using the tools we will teach you. Each chapter is followed by a set of questions. Readers can answer them in whatever form they'd like: discussion, writing (in the book or elsewhere), or they can simply ponder the questions.

Some kids may be mature enough to read this book on their own. Other kids will need their parent or another concerned adult to read it to them. You could even show this book to a counselor and see if they are willing and able to work on these principles with your child.

If you are a counselor who works with children who have been struck by the "I Feel Fat" Spell, you might try reading one chapter with them each session to give them time to absorb the lessons and integrate any changes in between sessions. Another option is to simply use some of the exercises as part of your therapy with them. You can also use this book as curriculum for a therapy group. Another option is to ask the parents to read it with their child at home.

For Kids:
Getting Started

If you spend a lot of time hating your body, trying to change certain body parts, and "feeling fat," you may have caught the "I Feel Fat" Spell. Hating your body is a painful way to live. And no matter what size you are, this book can help you feel better. In order to feel better, you have to learn how to change your *thinking*, not your body. This may not make sense to you right now, but we hope by the end of this book it will, and you will feel a whole lot better about yourself.

First, we have a little story for you called *The Mirror Witch*. This will give you a peek into what it's like to live in a world where kids feel comfortable in their bodies. You will also see what happens when kids get struck by the "I Feel Fat" Spell. Then, we have a bunch of new tools for you. We call them Spell Breakers. Spell Breakers take practice so when you find one that's helpful to you, stick with it for a while before going on to the next one.

If you have fallen under the "I Feel Fat" Spell, the good news is that the Spell Breakers in this book really work! We hope you will enjoy them, break free from the spell, and end up appreciating the body you live in.

The Mirror Witch

Once upon a time, there was a beautiful land where people of all colors, sizes, and shapes lived peacefully together. The people there were kind and helpful to one another, and the children lived and played without fear. They enjoyed and loved the bodies they were born with. They knew that all bodies were supposed to be different, just like all flowers, trees, and animals were unique. In this enchanted land, children loved food and ate just the right amount for their bodies when they were hungry. They loved to play, and they loved to rest. And they never compared themselves to anyone else.

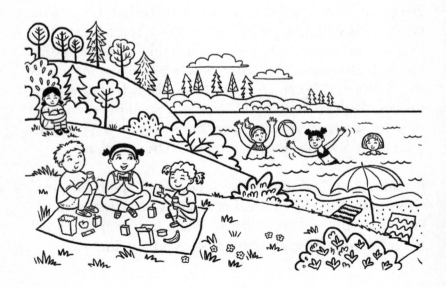

Whether they were tall or short, large or small, light-skinned or dark-skinned, all the children in the land felt lovable. They knew they were lovable, even when they were upset. They cried when they were sad and let out their anger when they were mad. They knew that if they let their feelings out when they felt them, they would soon feel peaceful again.

There were no mirrors in this land. The only places kids could see their reflections were in the beautiful lakes and ponds. They loved putting on their bathing suits and swimming all summer long. When they swam, the children could see themselves in the water, and it made them happy, no matter how they looked.

But one day, a mean witch showed up. She came because she was lonely. She had no friends because she was so mean. The witch decided that she would slip herself into

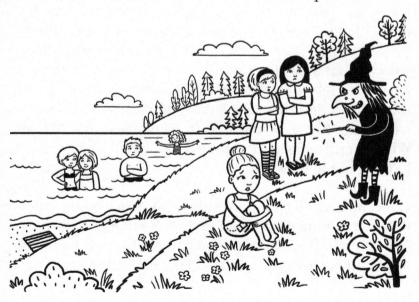

the water and make fun of the children. That way she wouldn't feel so alone. The children were so busy swimming and playing that they barely even noticed her. She didn't like that the children were ignoring her, and she knew she needed to come up with another way to get their attention.

This was right about the time the mirror was invented. So, the witch decided she would slip herself into all the mirrors and tease the children from there. This is how she became the **Mirror Witch**. When the children looked at themselves in the mirror, the **Mirror Witch** would say mean things to them like, "You're so fat," "You're ugly," or "Your thighs are too big."

Some kids completely ignored her because they knew she was just a mean witch. But other kids mistook her voice for their own thoughts. These kids believed what she was saying and eventually became possessed by the thoughts that the **Mirror Witch** planted inside of them. It was like they were under a spell. This spell made them worry about their size and compare themselves to others. These kids felt so bad and afraid that they returned to the mirror over and over to see if the **Mirror Witch's** insults were true. Some of these kids could hear the **Mirror Witch's** criticisms all the time, even when they weren't looking in the mirror.

Over time, more and more kids were struck by this spell. Worried parents took them to their Wellness Wizards to find out what was wrong. The parents learned their children had been struck by the "I Feel Fat" Spell.

Meanwhile, the **Mirror Witch** discovered that the more she convinced children to dislike their bodies, the more they would come back to the mirror and keep her company. So now, instead of playing, learning, dancing, and swimming, many of the children would stand in front of their mirrors, possessed by the spell that the witch had cast. She whispered to them about how their bodies weren't okay and how they should make themselves look better, telling them that if they followed her instructions, they would be liked and admired.

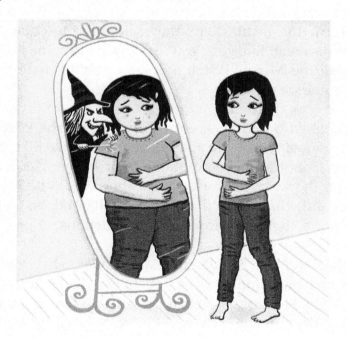

The **Mirror Witch** told each child they looked terrible no matter what they actually looked like. She told some kids they were too fat and others they were ugly. She told some kids to change their clothes again and again because they looked "fat in this shirt" and "terrible in those shorts." The more she insulted them, the longer they stood there and the less alone the **Mirror Witch** felt. She also told some kids to cut out certain foods or to eat as little as possible, and as they got thinner and weaker, they found it harder and harder to resist her spell.

Some children didn't fall under the **Mirror Witch's** spell. They were still playing with their friends, climbing trees, making crafts, and having picnics. These kids ate what their bodies needed to be strong and healthy. When the witch tried to insult them, they said, "I'm too busy for someone mean like you. You're no friend of mine." They ignored the **Mirror Witch** and kept playing with their real friends.

The kids who had been cursed by the **Mirror Witch's** spell wanted to feel free again. They didn't like that their whole lives had become about their body size. Even though the witch promised them they would be happy if they did what she said, they never felt good, no matter how perfectly they followed her instructions.

So, they went off in search of an answer. They looked high and low, under rocks and fallen trees. Suddenly, one of the kids found a beautiful ancient treasure chest, hidden deep inside a cave. When they lifted up the lid, to their surprise, they found twenty-two magical Spell Breakers. The instructions revealed that these Spell Breakers would help unhappy kids Reverse the Curse of the "I Feel Fat" Spell. It took them a while to master the Spell Breakers, but they did. Soon, they were out playing, swimming, and laughing with the other kids again and enjoying the beautiful world they lived in.

Can you figure out why some kids got caught by the "I Feel Fat" Spell and others didn't?

Do you think you have been caught by the spell?

If so, do you remember when you first felt like you were under the spell?

Spell Breakers

The children in our story caught the "I Feel Fat" Spell from the Mirror Witch, but in real life, children can catch the spell from many places, sort of like catching a cold or the flu. You were not born hating your body. You caught the "I Feel Fat" Spell and that caused you to start hating your body. And whether you caught it from someone at home or school, the computer, TV, or the movies, you can break the spell. That's where **Spell Breakers** come in. **Spell Breakers** will help you to Reverse the Curse.

Spell Breakers work the way medicine works when you're sick. The good news is that **Spell Breakers** don't taste gross like some medicines do. **Spell Breakers** change how you think, and they help you learn to like yourself. You might think that changing your body will help you like yourself, but the truth is, changing your *thinking* is what will help you. The first several **Spell Breakers** will teach you how to do this.

In the rest of the **Spell Breakers**, you will learn how to understand and break the "I Feel Fat" Spell. You will also learn lots of new ways to talk to yourself, how to become a stronger person, and how to let other people know what you feel and think.

Learning all of these things is important because the "I Feel Fat" Spell is about so much more than feeling fat. So, off we go, onto your very first **Spell Breaker**...

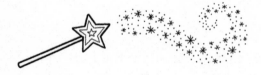

Spell Breaker #1:
Good Witch or Bad Witch?

When the Mirror Witch cast her spell on the kids in our story, it made them think she was their friend. They thought she was helping them by giving them important information that they needed to know like, "You're too big!" or "You're ugly!" and "No one likes you!" They didn't know the witch was lying to them and that she was just trying to get them to keep her company. Instead, they agreed with her that something was wrong with them. They even thought that their parents, who loved them more than they would ever know, were lying to them when they said, "There's nothing wrong with you!"

If anyone tried to get the kids to stop paying attention to the Mirror Witch, they would get mad. They thought she was a **Good Witch.** *She's my friend,* they would think. But their *real* friends knew she was a **Bad Witch.** Sometimes, their friends would say things like, "Don't be weird!" but that just made these kids want to hide their friendship with the witch. They were scared that without the Mirror Witch's advice, they wouldn't know what to do anymore or how to make themselves feel better.

The kids who believed that the Mirror Witch was their friend, forgot about all the trouble and pain she caused them. They didn't realize it was the Mirror Witch's fault that they hated their bodies. They didn't see that following her rules was causing problems with their parents, ruining the fun they used to have with their friends, and making them feel bad.

When the kids understood that the Mirror Witch was lying to them and causing them terrible pain, it then became possible for them to fight the witch and break her spell. They realized that the Mirror Witch was their problem, *not* their bodies. They started spending more time with their families and their real friends, instead of the witch.

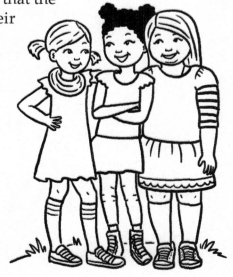

If you are one of the many children who also caught the "I Feel Fat" Spell and would like to break free, you are about to learn how to Reverse the Curse and feel free again. That's what all these Spell Breakers are about.

But before we get to the rest of the Spell Breakers, we want to let you know we understand that some of you might not *want* to break the spell. You might be afraid of what would happen if you did. That's normal. We have worked with many kids who were afraid to break the spell, and every single one of them is glad that they did.

*Do you think the Mirror Witch in the story is a **Good Witch** or a **Bad Witch**? Why?*

What might be hard about breaking the "I Feel Fat" Spell?

What do you think might be better in your life if you were free of the "I Feel Fat" Spell?

Spell Breaker #2: Unkind Mind—Kind Mind— Quiet Mind

In our Mirror Witch story, the witch cast a spell that made some children hate their bodies. But in real life, many kids have a voice in their head that sounds like the Mirror Witch but is really just their own minds talking to them in a mean way.

Did you know that your thoughts have the power to make your day a good one or a bad one? Having thoughts can be like having a dog. Sometimes we hang out and play with our dog. Sometimes we walk our dog peacefully down the street. Other times, the dog drags us down the street by its leash, barking at everyone! Well, sometimes

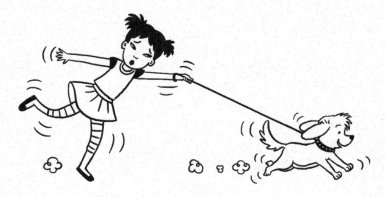

our minds can drag us around, just like an out-of-control dog. But a dog can be trained and so can our minds. We can train our minds to become more calm and kind.

Most kids don't realize that we have the power to change the mood of our minds. In this Spell Breaker, you will learn about three different mind moods: **Unkind Mind, Kind Mind, and Quiet Mind.**

First, let's look at a few examples of thoughts that an **Unkind Mind** has:

I'm too fat.
I'm ugly.
My nose is too big.
I'm stupid.
I can't do anything right.
Nobody likes me.
Everyone else is smarter than I am.
There's nothing special about me.

Sometimes (like when we fall under the "I Feel Fat" Spell), our minds can take over with really negative and mean thoughts like the examples above, and this can cause us to feel really unhappy.

Now let's look at a few examples of what a **Kind Mind** might sound like:

I don't have to be perfect.
I am special.
I am loveable no matter what my body looks like.

There are many good things about me.
I like my body. It helps me do so many
things I like to do.
If I practice something, I can become
better at it.

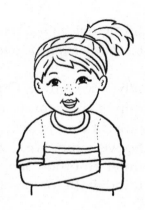

Spending more time in your **Kind Mind** will make you a happier person. But, if you have fallen under the "I Feel Fat" Spell, thoughts like these might seem impossible right now. If you hang in there and keep going with these Spell Breakers, **Kind Mind** will become easier to believe.

Finally, when you are in your **Quiet Mind**, you are not worrying about the past or the future. You're not focusing on what's negative or the things that scare you. You are just right where you are, using your five senses (sight, smell, touch, taste, and hearing) to notice what is around you.

Some examples of what it's like to have a **Quiet Mind** are:

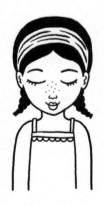

Sitting in a chair and noticing that the chair is brown. It's not good or bad, pretty or ugly; it's just brown.

Lying on the couch and noticing the feel of the cushion beneath you.

Feeling the soft grass under your feet when you are on the lawn or at the park.

Smelling dinner cooking in the kitchen.
Feeling the warm water when you are in the shower or the bath.

Taking time to really taste the food you are eating.
Listening to music without thinking about other things.

When we have a **Quiet Mind**, we are peaceful, and our minds are calm. It feels good. But when we get stuck in our **Unkind Mind,** it is not peaceful at all and definitely not very fun. We say mean things to ourselves and some-times to other people, too. A **Kind Mind** is a friendly mind, both to ourselves and to others.

*Most of the time, do you have a **Kind Mind, Unkind Mind,** or **Quiet Mind**?*

*What type of mind mood do you have right now? **Kind, Unkind, or Quiet**?*

*What are some of the things your **Unkind Mind** says?*

*What are some of the things your **Kind Mind** says?*

Spell Breaker #3: Beware—It's Unfair to Compare!

Your Unkind Mind gets you to compare yourself to other kids. But, **Beware—It's Unfair to Compare!** Usually, when people compare themselves to others, they don't make nice comparisons. Instead, they make mean comparisons and end up feeling bad about themselves.

Your Unkind Mind might say things like: *She's better at math than I am. He's better at soccer than I am. Those girls are skinnier than I am.* And you might agree, thinking, *That's right! I'm no good!* When you start thinking like this, a very good day can become a very bad day very quickly. You can start to feel like there's a dark cloud around you or like you suddenly gained a whole bunch of weight.

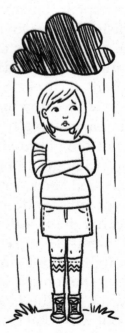

It's **Unfair to Compare** because when we compare ourselves to others, we are looking at them on the outside and thinking they must be happy or perfect on the inside. But all people have problems and difficulties, no matter what they look like.

Joanna was always comparing herself to the new girl at school named Olivia. Joanna was sure that because Olivia was really skinny, she must be perfect and really happy. Every time Joanna saw Olivia at school, Joanna felt horrible about her own body. She was sure that if she lost weight, she would be more confident and happy—just like she thought Olivia was. It took many months of feeling bad about herself before Joanna learned **It's Unfair to Compare.**

One day, she went over to Olivia's house after school. They spent some time doing homework and listening to music. Then, Olivia told Joanna all kinds of private things about her family and painful things that had happened to her before she moved to Joanna's town. Joanna was really surprised about how hard Olivia's life was. Her grandmother had just died, her parents were divorced, and her older brother had serious health problems. Boy, Joanna never thought about any of that when she compared herself to Olivia. All she ever thought about was what Olivia's body

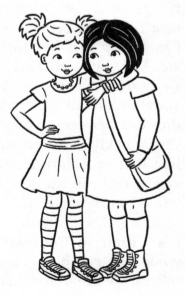

looked like. She was convinced that being skinny meant that Olivia had a perfect life. Joanna realized she would not want to trade her own life for Olivia's and that just because Olivia was thinner, it sure didn't mean she was happier!

Sometimes we feel like we are really different from others, and that being different is bad and makes us unlovable. It's true that we may have things about us that make us different, but it's *not* true that we are unlovable because of our differences. Our Unkind Mind tells us we should look and be exactly like other kids instead of like ourselves. But it's not a mistake that people look different. We›re supposed to be different! The world is made up of all kinds of people with all kinds of different talents and looks.

Think about nature, instead of people, for a minute. If you were to compare one tree to another tree, you probably wouldn't think, *Hmmm, that tree is skinnier than that other tree, so it's prettier.* Or if you saw a bunch of shells at the beach, you probably wouldn't say, "That shell is ugly because it's the only one with stripes." No, you would probably think that the striped shell is cool! Imagine a bucket of shells where every shell looks exactly the same. That's not nearly as interesting as a bucket with many different shapes and sizes of shells.

Imagine what a boring world it would be if there was only one type of tree, one kind of flower, or one type of shell. The same goes for people. We are not supposed to look or be the same. We all have differences that make us cool. Sometimes we can't see them because we are too busy listening to our Unkind Mind.

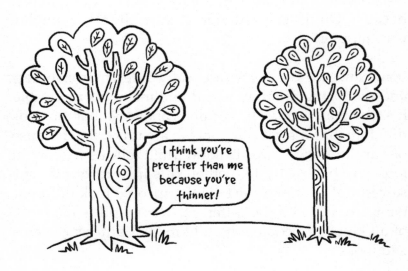

So, think of someone you compare yourself to. What does your Unkind Mind usually say when it compares the two of you? Try putting it in this sentence:

_____ is _____ than I am.
(Name of person)   (skinnier, prettier, smarter,
                          better, more popular)

Now, try taking out the Unfair Comparison, the most painful part of the sentence ("than I am"):

_____ is _____.
(For example: Suzie is skinny. Or Jennifer is pretty. Or Joey is smart.)

Now try saying both sentences again. Notice how different it feels to say it the second way, without the Unfair
Comparison. (The three little words "than I am" are what
makes comparisons so painful!) You don't have to allow
your Unkind Mind to make you feel bad just because
someone else has things about them that you like!

Sometimes people are smaller than we are, and sometimes
they are bigger, taller, shorter, darker, lighter, funnier,
smarter, or all kinds of other differences. This doesn't
mean that they, or we, are better or worse. And it doesn't
mean that they will have a better or worse life. Everybody
has some gifts and some problems, some things they are
good at, and some things they're not. So the next time
you catch yourself comparing, try taking away the Unfair
Comparison ("than I am"). You will be amazed at how
much better you feel.

Beware—It's Unfair to Compare!

*What are some of the topics you tend to make Unfair Comparisons
about (for example: number of friends, weight, appearance, grades)?*

*Do you think it's possible that the kids you compare yourself
to have things that make them sad, insecure, angry, or upset?*

Say three things that are good about you.

*Right now, tell your Unkind Mind, **"Beware—It's Unfair to
Compare!"***

Spell Breaker #4:
Bully or Buddy?

Most of the kids we work with are really kind and good to their friends. They tell us, "If a bully ever picked on my friend, I would protect them in a second. I would tell my friend to ignore that bully." These kids would never call their friends nasty names, but here are some of the things they say to themselves:

You're so fat!
You're a loser.
You're no good.

Now, doesn't that sound like a **Bully**? Did you know that you can be a **Bully** to yourself? You can be a **Bully** to yourself, or you can be a **Buddy**. A **Buddy** is friendly. A **Buddy** is kind. A **Buddy** doesn't tell you that you are a loser, and a **Buddy** doesn't call you mean names. Are you a **Bully** or a **Buddy** to yourself?

Remember The Mirror Witch? She was a **Bully**, and with her "I Feel Fat" Spell, she got the kids in the story to **Bully** themselves. In real life, kids often **Bully** themselves when they don't feel good inside. Some kids think that bullying themselves will help them to become better people. But, usually, it just makes them feel worse.

Some kids **Bully** themselves all day long. That's a horrible way to live! But kids can learn how to stop being a **Bully** to themselves and start being a **Buddy**.

Here are some different ways to become a better **Buddy** to yourself:

Sophia realized she was bullying herself, and she wanted to stop. She decided to be a **Buddy** to herself instead and think about all of the things that were good about her. One day, she made a list of all her good qualities and realized she was a really good friend and a good sister. She cared about animals, too. Thinking good things about herself made her feel so much better.

Riley decided to practice being a **Buddy**. Instead of saying mean things to himself in the mirror, he started smiling at himself when he saw his reflection.

Cody got sick and tired of his own inner **Bully**. He said to it, *You're a liar! I'm not going to listen to you anymore!*

Chloe started practicing being a **Buddy** to herself every time she heard her **Bully** voice. So when her **Bully** said *You're ugly,* she thought of what a **Buddy** would say and then said to herself, *You're not ugly, you're just feeling down right now.*

Gabby kept noticing her **Bully** voice at school. She learned that it made her feel really alone because other kids would be eating lunch together, and she would be lost in her Unkind Mind, listening to her **Bully**. She decided to say, *Knock it off. I am not that bad!* And then she joined the other kids for lunch.

*Do you have a **Bully** voice inside of you?*

*What are some things your **Bully** voice usually says to you?*

*Say something to yourself right now that a **Buddy** might say.*

Spell Breaker #5:
Retrain Your Brain

Many kids who are caught in the "I Feel Fat" Spell think they are unhappy mostly because of their bodies. But the truth is, they are mostly unhappy because of their thoughts. Of course, if our bodies are not healthy we can make positive changes to take better care of them, but in order to break the spell, we need to change our thinking.

Did you know that most human beings have about 70,000 thoughts a day? We think all day long. *Think, think, think.* Sometimes our thinking comes from Kind Mind and other times from Unkind Mind.

When you are in Quiet Mind, you think a little bit more slowly and calmly, and sometimes your mind is so quiet that you have no thoughts. Hopefully, someday, you will spend most of your time in Kind Mind and Quiet Mind and very little time in your Unkind Mind. In this Spell Breaker, we will be teaching you how to change some of your unkind thoughts into kind ones.

Have you ever seen a talking doll that has a recording inside of it? These toys usually have four or five things they repeat over and over. Well, that's how our minds can be. Sometimes we record a thought and we keep playing it over and over. With the dolls, it's usually something like, "I like you. You are my friend." But Unkind Mind records and plays things like, *I'm ugly*, or *My friend is better than me*, or *My stomach is gross*. Many kids believe these things, even if they're not true, because they believe their Unkind Mind no matter what it tells them. Well, the good news is, you can learn to delete these recordings and make new ones that feel so much better. When you do this, you **Retrain Your Brain**.

Learning to **Retrain Your Brain** is like learning anything new. It may not come easily at first, but with practice, you really can learn to change the way you think! So let's give it a try. Let's **Retrain Your Brain**!

Let's say your Unkind Mind is repeating *I'm too fat* over and over, and let's say you decide to **Retrain Your Brain**. The first step is to think of something nicer you can say to yourself. The **Retrain Your Brain** rule is that the new thought has to be something that's kind (or, at least, not unkind). So, using the example of *I'm too fat*, the new thought might be, *I'm lovable no matter what my size is*. (It's okay if you don't believe this new thought yet.)

The next step is to repeat the new thought to yourself a bunch of times, as many times a day as you can. The more the better! *I'm lovable no matter what my size is. I'm lovable no matter what my size is. I'm lovable no matter what my size is.*

The final step is to notice when you are thinking the old, unkind thought and immediately replace it with the new thought. So as soon as you hear yourself thinking, *I'm too fat,* you replace it with, *I'm lovable no matter what my size is.*

We know that your Unkind Mind may not like this at all. It might try to convince you that the kind thought is wrong or untrue. It might disagree, argue, or it might even shout louder to try to drown out the new thought. That's okay. Just keep repeating the kind thought as much as you can. Over time, the Unkind Mind will give up. You *can* **Retrain Your Brain**.

Can you think of any reasons that you wouldn't want to spend more time in your Kind Mind or Quiet Mind?

Think of a new kind thought you would like to have. Now repeat it to yourself at least five times. How did that feel?

How did your Unkind Mind react to your new thought?

Spell Breaker #6:
Strong, Soft, Silly, or Silent

We all talk to ourselves all day long. We don't usually do this out loud, but inside our heads we have thoughts going on all the time. As you've been learning in some of the other Spell Breakers, some of our thoughts are kind, and some are not so kind. In the case of the "I Feel Fat" Spell, some people's thoughts are just plain mean.

Once you realize that your Unkind Mind is doing too much of the talking, and you want to stop it, you will learn that there are many ways to do that. In this Spell Breaker, we will teach you four ways: **Strong, Soft, Silly, or Silent**.

If your sister, brother, or friend was annoying you, you might ask them to stop in a **Strong** voice, or you might ask them to stop in a **Soft**, kind voice. You might decide to be **Silly**, to joke around with them and not take them too seriously. Or you might even decide to be **Silent** and just ignore them.

Some children talk back to their "I Feel Fat" voice or their Unkind Mind in a **Strong** way. So when their Unkind Mind tells them they are too fat, they say things back to it like, *Leave me alone. You are mean. You are a bully!* Talking back like this helps them feel **Strong** inside.

Other kids talk back to their Unkind Mind in a **Soft** way such as, *Please be quiet. I am a good person, and I just want to be free to live my life.* Or, *I know you are trying to help me, but you're really not.* This helps them to quiet their Unkind Mind and feel more peaceful.

Another way to handle the Unkind Mind is to be playful or **Silly**. So, for example, if your Unkind Mind says, *Nobody likes you,* you can repeat that right back in a really **Silly** voice: *Nobody likes YOU!* Or you could put your fingers in your ears and say, *I'm not listening!* Or you could simply say, *Whatever!* The Unkind Mind will realize you're not taking it seriously and will get quieter or may even go away completely.

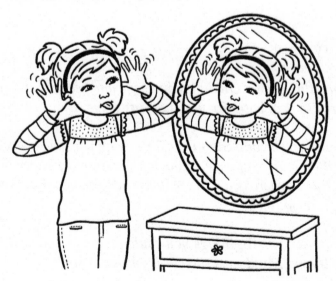

The fourth way of dealing with your Unkind Mind is to be **Silent** and ignore it. This means you just go on with your day and think about other things.

As you can see, there are lots of different things you can say or do to respond to your Unkind Mind. The important thing is to figure out what helps *your* mind become peaceful. You can experiment with **Strong, Soft, Silly, or Silent** and see what works best for you.

So, let's look at all the options. If your Unkind Mind says, *You are ugly,* you can reply in a **Strong** way like, *I'm just fine, YOU are NO GOOD!* Or you can talk back in a **Soft** way like, *Leave me alone, please. I'm busy.* You can try being **Silly.** You can dance around, make funny faces in the mirror, or turn what the Unkind Mind is saying into a **Silly** song. Or, you can just stay **Silent,** totally ignore it and go play with a friend, or do something else you like to do.

Let's try it out...

*Pick one thing your Unkind Mind says and see how it feels to talk back to it in both **Strong** and **Soft** ways.*

*Now, pick one helpful **Strong** or **Soft** thing you said above and write it on a piece of paper. You can decorate the paper if you want. Put it where you will see it everyday so you don't forget to say it to yourself.*

*What are some **Silly** things you could do or say the next time your Unkind Mind says something mean to you?*

What are some things you can do when you want to simply ignore the Unkind Mind?

Spell Breaker #7:
Dog Talk or Cat Chat

Kids who have been struck by the "I Feel Fat" Spell have a hard time speaking kindly to themselves. When we ask these kids what they think about themselves or their bodies, they sometimes sound like the meanest kids on earth. But ask one of these kids how she feels about her dog (or cat), and she is suddenly the kindest kid around! If you, too, are mean to yourself and think unkind thoughts about your body, here is another way you can learn how to speak more kindly to yourself. We call it **Dog Talk or Cat Chat** depending on which animal you like better.

Dog Talk and **Cat Chat** are when you talk to yourself in the same sweet, loving voice that you use to talk to a dog or cat that you love. (If you don't like dogs or cats, you can think of another animal that you love. If you're not an animal lover, you can think about a baby or a young child.) When we ask kids to tell us how they feel when they think of their favorite pet, or a little baby, their faces light up. They feel love, and this usually fills them with happy thoughts.

Sadly, many kids treat their pets way better than they treat themselves. If your dog had a roll on her tummy would you call her mean names and hate her? Of course not! But do you do that to yourself? If another cat hissed at your cat, would you think your cat was unlovable or needed to lose weight? No way! But do you think you're unlovable or need to lose weight when someone is angry with you? These are things kids think about themselves when they are caught in the "I Feel Fat" Spell. Not only do they treat their pets way better than they treat themselves, but many kids are especially mean to themselves when they are down, even though this is when they need kindness the most.

How would you treat your special pet or a child if they were hurt or feeling down? How would you treat them if they were tired or hungry? If a dog was whining for food, would you ever in a million years think of letting it go hungry? If your kitty wasn't feeling well, would you tell him he was a loser? Do you do that to yourself? Well, if you know how to love a pet or your family and friends, you can learn to love yourself!

Think about the way you speak to a precious animal, baby or young child. Notice how your voice sounds. You probably use your sweetest voice. We bet you are understanding and kind. You might say things like, "I love you!" "You're so cute!" "Come here and play!"

Let's try a little experiment. Think of an animal (or a baby) that you really love. Think about all the things you love about it and how you feel when you see how cute and precious it is. Inside your head, say something sweet to it and notice what your voice sounds like. Pay attention to where you feel the love in your body. Is it in your heart, stomach, or chest? Maybe you feel it all over your body. See if you can let that feeling get even bigger inside of you. (Funny how the animal might not even be with you right now, but you can still feel the love.) Now imagine looking at your body with the same love you feel for that precious pet. Say something sweet to your body in the same voice you used for the pet. If you can't think of something, try, *I love you, amazing body!*

Dog Talk and **Cat Chat** are great ways to speak to yourself, especially when you are feeling down. Don't worry if you can't do it yet. You can try again tomorrow—and the day after that! We usually don't get good at things unless we practice, so you can practice **Dog Talk or Cat Chat** until you get good at it!

What sweet things do you usually say when you're talking to your favorite animal?

Pick one and say it to yourself right now. See how that feels.

Spell Breaker #8:
Getting to the Root

You were not born feeling bad about your body. Babies live in their bodies without any thoughts or worries about what they look like. They are simply present.

There are important reasons why kids start to hate their bodies. Thinking about what started your "I Feel Fat" Spell is what we call **Getting to the Root**. It's like pulling a weed from the garden. To get rid of a weed, you have to go deep into the soil and make sure you pull it all the way out, including the root, otherwise it will just grow right back.

So, let's try **Getting to the Root** of what might have started your bad body thoughts. Here are some things kids have told us about why they started to "feel fat." See if you relate to any of these for yourself:

1. My brother teased me about my thighs and I felt so embarrassed.

2. I overheard my mom criticizing her body. Everyone tells me I look like her.

3. My friends at school talk about how fat they feel but I'm bigger than they are.

4. My dad told me I was eating too much.

5. My gym teacher said I'd be a faster runner if I lost a little weight.

6. My favorite singers look so thin and happy, so I thought I would be happier if I looked more like them.

7. I gained weight over the summer and people teased me about it.

It's so easy for kids to think their problem is simply their bodies. But the real problem is *why* they started hating their bodies in the first place. It's kind of like if something was wrong with your computer, you couldn't fix it by just getting a new screen. You would have to get help finding out what was wrong inside of it.

So, let's start **Getting to the Root** of *your* "I Feel Fat" Spell.

Do any of the things in the list above sound like something that happened to you?

What are your earliest memories of not liking certain parts your body of your body? (It's okay if you don't know right now, maybe you'll remember later.)

What emotions did you feel when that happened?

Spell Breaker #9: Follow the Clues

Have you ever had a time when one minute you felt okay in your body and then *something happened*, and the next minute you suddenly felt like you gained a bunch of weight? How can that be? Your body didn't magically change and gain twenty pounds in two seconds! What happened was that your Kind Mind, or your Quiet Mind, suddenly turned into an Unkind Mind. And the weirdest part is that once you started focusing on what your Unkind Mind said, you forgot that *something happened* that made you switch to an Unkind Mind.

Here are some examples of things that can get the Unkind Mind started:

Someone teasing you
Thinking of something that makes you sad or mad
Feeling nervous or scared about something
Feeling lonely or bored

Lots of times, these painful things happen to kids, but they skip right over dealing with them, and instead they start thinking they are too fat. So, we can use our unkind thoughts as clues, like a detective would, to help us discover what happened. Instead of listening to the mean things that our Unkind Mind tells us, we can notice *when* our minds get unkind and ask ourselves, "What just happened?" Then we can think about whether it was something we thought, saw, or heard that made us feel uncomfortable. This is how you **Follow the Clues.** It's important to **Follow the Clues** because then you can solve your *real* problems instead of being tricked by the Unkind Mind into focusing on your body.

Alyssa **Followed the Clues** and realized she was upset because someone had teased her. Instead of feeling upset about getting teased, her Unkind Mind popped up with the thought that she was fat and ugly.

Cody noticed his Unkind Mind was yelling at him like crazy. He used this as a clue that something else was going on. After thinking about when it started, he realized it was shortly after he discovered that his bike had been stolen. He wasn't "dumb" like his Unkind Mind was telling him. He was angry that someone had stolen his bike.

Brooke said her Unkind Mind was talking ALL the time. (This made it difficult to figure out where to look for clues.) Her unkind mind told her she had fat thighs and ugly eyes and gross hair and all kinds of other horrible things. While speaking to a counselor, she realized that she was sad all the time because her parents had just divorced, and that's why her Unkind Mind seemed endless. She didn't even realize she was sad because she was so busy listening to her Unkind Mind! The counselor helped her **Follow the Clues.**

So, the next time your Unkind Mind gets loud, see if you can **Follow the Clues** and figure out what is really going on. If you get stuck, it can help to talk to someone you trust. When you fall under a spell, your mind is actually tricking you, which can make it difficult to see that there are clues. Other people can help you **Follow the Clues** when you have difficulty doing it yourself.

What are some of the things your Unkind Mind says that can remind you it's time to ***Follow the Clues?***

Name three things you are sad or mad about that have nothing to do with your body.

Who can you trust to talk to about things that are painful for you?

Spell Breaker #10: Mind Movies or Really Real

Here is a secret that will help you throughout your whole life. Ready?

Thoughts are not real! They *feel* real, but they aren't real. They can make us very sad sometimes, or ashamed, scared, or hurt, but still, the thoughts in our minds are not real.

Think about it. Can you pull one single thought out of your mind and show it to somebody? Can you fold a thought up and put it in your pocket? The answer is "no" because your thoughts are not real! They are kind of like movies that play in your mind. We call them **Mind Movies**. Many people forget that their thoughts are just **Mind Movies** and, instead, think that their thoughts are **Really Real**.

For example, when you watch a movie on TV, you know the movie is not real life, right? It's a movie. The couch you're sitting on is real, the person next to you is real, if you're eating snacks, those are real, but the story isn't really happening it's just a movie. It's not **Really Real**.

Another example is when you wake up from a nightmare. Hopefully you know the nightmare wasn't real. But your bed is real, and the pillow is real. Can you see the difference between **Really Real** and **Mind Movies**?

So what is **Really Real**? We're glad you asked!

If you can see it, smell it, feel it, taste it, touch it, or hear it, it's real. If it's in your head, it's just a thought, or a **Mind Movie**, and it may be true or it may be false, but it isn't **Really Real**.

Brianna was in the car with her mom. She looked out the window and saw her friend, Emily, in the next car with her family. Brianna waved, but Emily didn't wave back. Then a **Mind Movie** started in Brianna's brain. In this **Mind Movie**, Emily was mad at her and told all their friends bad things about Brianna. Then her friends turned on her, and no one wanted to hang out with her anymore. This scary movie played inside Brianna's mind while she rode home with her mom. By the time she got home, she was in a very bad mood.

But, wait! Brianna suddenly remembered that this was just a **Mind Movie**. It wasn't **Really Real**. It didn't really happen! The only thing that was **Really Real** was that she was in the car with her mom, and she waved to her friend and her friend didn't wave back. So, she called Emily on the phone. She asked, "Did you see me? I just drove by you in the car!" Emily said, "Where? When? I didn't even see you!" And they talked for a while and said they would see each other at school the next day. Phew! It was all just a **Mind Movie**!

Once you know about **Mind Movies**, there's a really cool thing you can do: Change the Channel. All you have to do is think about something else! It's like when you are watching TV, and you decide to watch something different. If you're watching a scary movie, or something that you don't like, you can Change the Channel to something else. Well, you can learn how to do the same thing with your mind.

When you realize you are in a **Mind Movie**, you can sing a song, take five deep breaths and count them as you go, or think about something you like. Or you can get **Really Real** and focus on what is really around you, like what you see with your eyes. Or the sounds you hear. Or what you feel with your hands and feet. Anytime you catch yourself in a **Mind Movie**, you can bring yourself back to what is **Really Real**. Changing the Channel can make you feel a lot better than watching a scary **Mind Movie**.

Lila caught herself in a **Mind Movie** when she was in the bathtub. Lila spent most of her bath time thinking unkind things about her body. Instead of enjoying her bath, she got lost in a **Mind Movie** that sounded something like, *My thighs are so fat and my arms are so gross. No one will ever like someone like me.* When she learned about **Mind Movies**, she began to Change the Channel and bring herself back to what was **Really Real**. So instead of letting her **Mind Movies** ruin her bath, she began to focus on the warm water, the sudsy bath bubbles, and the sweet smell of her favorite shampoo. When Lila learned to Change the Channel, her bath time went from being a hard time to a sweet, quiet time. She said, "It's like watching something on the 'I Feel Fat-elodoen' channel and then changing it to a much better show."

When kids think that **Mind Movies** are **Really Real**, they can do all kinds of strange things. They can stop talking to a friend because their **Mind Movie** was about their friend not liking them. They can try to starve themselves because their **Mind Movie** was about being too big. They can exercise too much because their **Mind Movie** was about being more popular if they had more muscles.

When you learn how to stop believing your **Mind Movies** and how to Change the Channel, you will live in what is **Really Real,** and it is a much better place to live.

Melissa made up a cool way to experience what is **Really Real** instead of stressing out on **Mind Movies.** While she walked around, she would think to herself, *Feel the ground, hear a sound, notice what is all around.* Doing this over and over took her mind off negative movies and helped her relax and feel better.

*Look around you. What is one **Really Real** thing you can see right now? What is one **Really Real** thing you can hear right now? What is one **Really Real** thing your body is touching right now?*

*Now, see if you can notice the difference between what is **Really Real** and the thoughts in your mind.*

Spell Breaker #11:
Fat is Not a Feeling!

You may have heard the sentence, "I feel fat." You may even say it to yourself sometimes (or a lot). You might even say it out loud. Maybe you've even heard some of the adults in your life say it. But guess what? **Fat is NOT a Feeling!** So, if **Fat is Not a Feeling**, then what is a feeling?

Feelings are natural human reactions that happen inside all of us. Usually they are described with only one word. Some feelings are pleasant, like happy, glad, and peaceful. Other feelings are more painful like scared, sad, and mad. But all feelings are important, natural, and part of being alive.

Here are some common feelings:
(Notice that "fat" isn't one of them!)

Happy   Guilty

Mad   Sad

Lonely   Scared

Healthy kids have a good relationship with their feelings. They don't think some feelings are "bad," or that they shouldn't be felt or talked about. They know that all feelings are important and need to be allowed. It's kind of like when we have to go to the bathroom, we just know we need to go, and it doesn't do any good to pretend we don't or to try to make that feeling go away. So when we feel sad, we need to talk about it and let our tears out. When we are angry, scared, or embarrassed, we need to talk about those feelings, too.

Our feelings go up and down all the time. It's sort of like riding a roller coaster. One minute you might be happy and another minute you might be really sad. You might feel excited about something new and then feel really scared about it. Or you might have a bunch of different feelings at the same time. All of this is a normal part of being alive.

One thing that helps us ride the roller coaster of feelings is to remember that feelings go up and down for everyone. Another thing that helps is to know what to hold on to when the ride gets bumpy or scary. Talking to or hugging someone we trust, writing in a journal, or telling ourselves something really comforting are some of the ways to hold on when the ride gets difficult. We can also hold onto something comforting like a favorite blanket, a stuffed animal, or a pet.

Feelings live in your body, and when you let them out, they eventually calm down. So if you feel sad and you let yourself cry, the sadness will pass, and then you won't feel sad anymore (until the next time you feel sad about something). That's how it works. But a lot of people think that they need to hold their feelings inside, and this causes them to feel very unhappy and alone.

So how did it come to be that so many people say, "I feel fat" when **Fat is Not a Feeling**? How did "fat" get on the list of feelings?

We live in a really busy world where most people have their heads in iPads, cell phones, or computers on top of school, homework, and everything else. Sometimes people get so busy that they forget to pay attention to what they are feeling inside. But we all have a really important world inside of us (our feelings), and this inner world needs attention. With so much focus on the outside world of doing things, getting things, and changing how they look, many people don't even know what they feel inside. When they think about how they feel, they focus on the outside, rather than the inside. They say, "I feel fat" instead of, "I feel mad" (or sad, scared, or bored).

Plus, on top of that, the messages we get from TV and the computer tell us we are supposed to be really skinny and never get fat. This makes many people worry about being fat. Then they talk about feeling fat, rather than feeling worried. And every time they feel worried, they think it's because they are fat (whether they are fat or not!) This is an example of mixing up feelings with fat, even though **Fat is Not a Feeling!**

If you are someone who thinks, or says, "I feel fat," this might really mean you don't feel good about yourself. "I feel fat" could mean you feel *scared* because you think you're not okay. It could mean you feel *upset* that you don't look like the people in magazines, in movies, or on the Internet. Or you might be feeling *anxious* that you don't look the same as some of your friends. So, when you say, "I feel fat," you might really mean, "I feel scared," or "I feel upset," or "I feel anxious." Scared, upset, and anxious are feelings. But, **Fat is Not a Feeling!**

So, if **Fat is Not a Feeling,** then what is it?

Fat is the soft part of our bodies. Everybody has and needs fat. Our bodies need fat in order to function. Fat keeps us warm. It protects our organs like a pillow, and it cushions our bones. Can you imagine sitting on a wooden chair with no fat for a cushion? Ouch!

Fat is also an important food group. Our bodies store fat to use for energy. Fat adds flavor to our food so it tastes really yummy! And it helps keep us from getting hungry too soon after eating. So, as you can see, fat is important. And one thing is for sure, **Fat is Not a Feeling!**

Do you remember how to Follow the Clues? Well, every time you say, "I feel fat," you have a clue to follow. You can think about what happened right before you had that thought. Was there a real feeling that you missed?

What three feelings are you feeling right now? (Look at the feelings in the beginning of this Spell Breaker if you get stuck.)

Try to remember the last time you thought or said, "I feel fat." What do you think you were really feeling?

What are some ways you can get comfort when you are having painful feelings?

Spell Breaker #12: Fat Chat Is Not Where It's At!

Imagine living in a world where everyone was happy with the body they were born with! Sadly, we don't. There are many people who don't feel good about their bodies. So, there is a very good chance you have heard what we call **"Fat Chat."**

Fat Chat is when people say mean things about how they or others look. It's also **Fat Chat** when people talk in public about needing to lose weight. Diet talk is **Fat Chat**, too. Even positive comments about bodies can be **Fat Chat** because of the focus on looks, which creates pressure to look a certain way.

Here are some examples of **Fat Chat**:

"She's so skinny!"

"I'm not going to eat that; it's fattening."

"She's so good because she's exercising a lot."

"Does this make me look fat?"

"He has a perfect body."

"Wow, look how much she's eating!"

Many people do **Fat Chat** because it helps them feel like they are part of a group or are better than others. But what **Fat Chat** really does is hurt people. It hurts the people that are being talked about, and it hurts everyone who is listening because **Fat Chat** can make us feel like we have to be perfect so we won't get talked about, too.

Fat Chat Is Not Where It's At!

Now, we might not be able to stop other people from doing **Fat Chat,** but we can definitely stop doing it ourselves! We know it's not always easy to be different from the crowd. Sometimes it seems easier to follow along with what other people are doing. So, if people around you are doing **Fat Chat,** it can take a lot of courage to disagree or ask them to stop. You would have to be a leader instead of a follower. But you can choose to be different than other people and not just go along with the crowd.

There are people that don't like cats, but if you are a cat-lover, you don't have to agree with what they think. There are people that say mean things about other groups of people, and you don't have to agree with that either. You can think and act differently.

So, when people are doing **Fat Chat,** you don't have to agree that skinnier is better or that dieting is good for you. If someone makes fun of someone's body, you don't have to join in. If you don't feel comfortable or brave enough to disagree out loud, you could just stay silent. **Fat Chat Is Not Where It's At!**

Here are some ways you can stop **Fat Chat**:

Tell people what **Fat Chat** is and ask them to try not to do it.

When people are doing **Fat Chat** say, "I'm uncomfortable with this kind of talk," or, "That's not very nice."

You can stay silent while people are **Fat Chatting** and remind yourself that **Fat Chat Is Not Where It's At!**

When you hear someone say something unkind about someone else's body, you can say, "I think she (or he) is fine just the way they are."

If someone makes a joke about the size or shape of someone else's body, don't laugh.

Tell the **Fat Chatters**, "I'm really trying not to talk so much about weight and food anymore."

If someone is talking about some food being bad, or fattening, you can say, or think, "I love this food. A medium-sized amount is fine."

So the next time you catch yourself wanting to **Fat Chat** about someone else, stop yourself and say something kind about that person instead (or say nothing at all).

And the next time you want to do **Fat Chat** on yourself (like, *I'm so fat* or *My thighs are huge*), see if you can stop yourself and say something nice. Or, simply notice what you are feeling. (Remember to Follow the Clues!)

Fat Chat Is Not Where It's At!

Does anyone in your life do **Fat Chat***?*

What can you do the next time you hear **Fat Chat***?*

What is one thing you can say or think when you are wanting to **Fat Chat** *about yourself or someone else?*

Spell Breaker #13:
Slip 'n Slide

Have you ever played on a **Slip 'n Slide**? The water on the plastic makes it super slippery and you can slide away really fast! Well, here's a cool Spell Breaker that uses your imagination. We call it **Slip 'n Slide**! **Slip 'n Slide** is a way to protect yourself from hurtful things that can happen with other people and not let every mean thing go straight into you, like a "Dart in the Heart."

Unless you live on an island all by yourself, you have to deal with people every day. And sometimes these people are going to say or do things that feel painful to you. For example, people might tease you, or they might purposely, or accidentally, say something that hurts you. Or you might hear something (that wasn't said to you) that makes you feel bad.

When kids feel bad about themselves, they let mean comments go straight into their hearts, and that's why the comments hurt so badly. But when kids decide to **Slip 'n Slide**, the mean words people say don't become a Dart in the Heart; they simply **Slip 'n Slide** right off them.

You can also picture mean words bouncing or flying away. These are **Slip 'n Slides**, too. There are lots of different ways to **Slip 'n Slide**. Here are some examples:

*If someone says something mean to you, you can pretend you are covered in water and let the comment **Slip 'n Slide** right off you.*

*Picture a big bucket in between you and the person being mean to you and imagine that what they are saying is **Slip 'n Sliding** right into the bucket and not into your heart or your mind!*

If somebody says something unkind about your body, you can picture a big bubble around you so that what they say doesn't even touch you. It bounces right off!

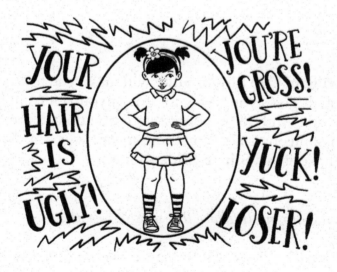

Imagine a wall between you and a bully and picture the mean things the bully says bouncing off the wall.

Picture yourself blowing your painful feelings into balloons and then watch the balloons fly away.

Imagine that you have a protective shield in front of you so that mean things just bounce off it.

Pretend that you can throw mean words into an imaginary fire and watch them burn up.

While watching TV or looking at the computer, imagine a shield in front of you that protects you from any Fat Chat before it hits you.

*Make up your own way to **Slip 'n Slide**! Describe it here:*

Knowing how to **Slip 'n Slide** will make you a stronger person. It gives you a way to protect yourself from hurtful words. And don't worry if you can't do it at the time when someone says something mean, you can always imagine doing a **Slip 'n Slide** later on.

*Pick one **Slip 'n Slide** idea that you like the best.*

Think about a time when someone said something that hurt you.

*Now, imagine using your favorite **Slip 'n Slide** with that hurtful memory and see how it feels.*

Spell Breaker #74: Stick to the Facts

Do you know the difference between facts and thoughts? A fact is something that anyone can see. It's Really Real. A thought is a personal opinion. A bunch of thoughts together make a Mind Movie. Sometimes people have the same thoughts or opinions as someone else, and sometimes they don't.

There is a big difference between facts and thoughts. Here are some examples:

Fact: This chair is brown.
Thought: This chair is ugly.

Fact: Abigail got a higher grade than I did in Math class.
Thought: I'm dumb.

Fact: Jasmine is skinny.
Thought: Jasmine has a perfect life.

Can you tell the difference between the facts and the thoughts?

Can you see that some thoughts can be very wrong? They are not facts. A fact is the truth. It is something that happened, is happening right in front of you, or is definitely true. A thought is made up. We may believe it, but that doesn't mean it's true. It's not definite. It's a personal opinion. Some people think a brown chair is ugly, some think a brown chair is pretty, but either way, it's brown and it's a chair. Brown and chair are the facts. Ugly and pretty are the thoughts.

Some people go around all day thinking, *I am good,* or *I am bad. She's a jerk,* or *She is better than me. He's a loser,* or *He's cool.* These are all thoughts, not facts.

When kids are struck by the "I Feel Fat" Spell, they usually believe the negative thoughts they have about themselves and think those thoughts are facts, when in fact, they are just thoughts! Believing that negative thoughts are facts, is a big cause of unhappiness. When we are in our Unkind Mind, we can go from one negative thought to the next, and this makes us feel worse and worse. Especially when we believe everything we think. But, when we **Stick to the Facts,** we feel so much better than when we stick to our thoughts!

Here's how it works: Let's say you have a friend with curly hair. Instead of thinking her hair is pretty or ugly, you can **Stick to the Facts** and think to yourself, *Her hair is curly.* Or, if somebody cries, instead of thinking they are a crybaby, you can **Stick to the Facts** and think, *They are upset right now.*

It can be a little easier to **Stick to the Facts** when it's about something or someone else, but now let's see how to **Stick to the Facts** when it's about you. The next time you look in the mirror, see if you can **Stick to the Facts**. Look at the facts only, and say things like, "I see a red shirt, brown hair, the skin on my arms, a nose, and two eyes." The next time you look down at your body, try to **Stick to the Facts**. "I see blue pants, brown shoes, and a little bit of my socks."

Now you have another way of breaking the "I Feel Fat" Spell. Instead of listening to your Unkind Mind, you can **Stick to the Facts.**

Look around you right now and find five facts.

Now to really challenge yourself, look in a mirror and find three facts about your body.

*As you go through your day, see how much you can **Stick to the Facts**.*

Spell Breaker #15: Say What You Mean but Don't Say It Mean

Children learn a lot of different subjects in school, but one really important thing that's not usually taught is how to talk about difficult feelings. It's pretty easy to say nice things to other people like, "That's a cool shirt," or "Good catch at the game," or "I had so much fun at your party." But what about the hard things? What about when someone hurts your feelings or when someone is doing something that you don't like? These things can be really hard to talk about. That's when you need to **Say What You Mean but Don't Say It Mean**.

A lot of people, even grownups, don't know how to **Say What You Mean but Don't Say It Mean**. When they don't know how, they sometimes end up saying mean things or not saying anything at all.

When somebody hurts your feelings, it can be really easy to say something mean like, "You're a jerk!" instead of something not mean like, "That hurt my feelings." Or if you feel really bad about something, it can be easy to say nothing at all, hide your feelings, and sometimes even think that you are bad and that's why somebody hurt you. The better thing to do would be to find someone you trust and tell them about what happened and why you feel hurt. They can help you with the problem and remind you that you're not bad.

When people don't let out their feelings, their feelings stay stuffed down inside of them. This can make them feel uncomfortable because feelings need to be let out. Many people find that when they don't talk about their feelings, they end up thinking they are too big because their feelings are all stuffed inside of them. (They are having BIG feelings!)

So, one way to stop "feeling fat" is to **Say What You Mean but Don't Say It Mean**. This means finding a calm, kind, and mature way to tell someone how you feel. We will teach you how to do that.

First, think about a time when someone did something you really didn't like. Complete the following sentence remembering to Stick to the Facts.

"When you _____"

Here are some examples:

1. *When you turned off the light while I was still in the room...*

2. *When you borrowed my shirt without asking...*

3. *When you put mustard on my hot dog...*

The next step is to add what you felt. Try to use one or two feelings.

1. When you turned off the light while I was still in the room, *I felt scared.*

2. When you borrowed my shirt without asking, *I felt mad and frustrated.*

3. When you put mustard on my hot dog, *I felt disgusted and upset.*

The last step is to add what you do or don't want:

1. When you turned off the light while I was still in the room, I felt scared. *Could you remember that I'm scared of the dark and be careful not to turn the light off when I'm in the room?*

2. When you borrowed my shirt without asking, I felt mad and frustrated. *Could you ask me first when you want to borrow something?*

3. When you put mustard on my hot dog, I felt disgusted and upset. *Could you try to remember that I really don't like mustard?*

So that's it! If you can learn to **Say What You Mean but Don't Say It Mean**, you won't have to either be mean to people or stuff your feelings down.

One last thing to keep in mind is that even when you say something in a kind way, there may be times that other people don't have the best reactions. If that happens, you can still be proud that you did your best to **Say What You Mean but Don't Say It Mean.**

What is one thing that you have been feeling hurt or mad about?

Now, try putting that example in the first blank below. Then, fill in the second blank with one or two feelings, and the third blank with a request.

When you _____,
I felt _____.
Could you _____?

Now you know how to **Say What You Mean but Don't Say It Mean.**

Spell Breaker #16: Just Say Yes!

You may not remember the first time you ever said the word "no" but it was probably one of the very first words you ever spoke. Being able to say "no" is very important because we need to be able to tell others what we don't want. For example, we might not want to go to a friend's house. We might not want chips with our sandwich. We might not be ready to go to sleep yet. Of course, some things we won't have a choice about. For example, it's fine if we say "no" to eating peas, but it's not fine if we say "no" to *all* vegetables. Or it could be fine if we don't want to go to sleep right away, but it's not fine if we want to stay up so late that we can't get up for school in the morning!

One of the things that can make our lives much more peaceful is understanding what things to say "no" to and what things to say "yes" to. Saying "no" to our height or the color of our eyes will not help us because we can't change our height or eye color. Saying "no" to the things we can't change just ends up making us feel unhappy. When tall people can accept the fact that they are tall, and even find what might be good about it, they will be much happier than if they hate being tall. Whether someone says "yes" to being tall or "no" to it, they are still tall. The difference is that saying "yes" will make them feel more peaceful. So, sometimes we need to **Just Say Yes**.

When kids are struck with the "I Feel Fat" Spell, they spend a lot of time saying "no" to parts of their bodies. Of course, this doesn't change their bodies, it just makes them feel miserable. Sometimes they become so miserable they do really unhealthy things to try to change their bodies. This can cause many problems over time. The truth is, all bodies are different, meaning that everybody has a one-of-a-kind body. And all bodies change over time as we grow up and age. Bodies are not like boxes that stay exactly the same size. And bodies are not like clay that we can mold. Human bodies change and grow as we change and grow. Our job is to take really good care of them and **Just Say Yes**.

Just like all bodies are different, all personalities are different, too. Some of us are shy, and some of us are talkative. We are *supposed* to be different from one another.

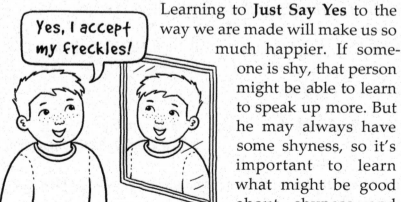

Learning to **Just Say Yes** to the way we are made will make us so much happier. If someone is shy, that person might be able to learn to speak up more. But he may always have some shyness, so it's important to learn what might be good about shyness and what strengths he has as a person. If he doesn't learn to **Just Say Yes** to the type of personality he has, he will be pretty unhappy. When we can accept and find the good things about being tall or short or shy or talkative, we will be so much happier.

If you **Just Say Yes**, that doesn't mean you can't make changes. Some people with curly hair will straighten their hair and some people with straight hair will curl it! But for the most part, we all have our unique shapes and sizes. We can spend our lives hating them, being miserable and trying to change them, or we can learn to accept what we were born with, **Just Say Yes,** and live a much more peaceful life.

Kids who **Just Say Yes** to the things they can't change feel so much better than kids who always want to change themselves. So let's try out both ways and see how they feel to you.

Think of one body part that's impossible to change.

See what it feels like to say, "No! I will NOT accept my
_____.*"*
(use body part from above)

Now see what it feels like to say, "Yes! I accept my _____."
(use body part from above)

Try repeating this statement to yourself three times. How does that feel?

Spell Breaker #17: Strong as a Tree or Wiggly as a Weed

Imagine what happens when a big wind blows against a tall, sturdy tree. Now imagine what happens when a big wind blows against a tiny, little weed. The tree stands strong but the weed wiggles all around.

When kids feel good about who they are, and are strong on the inside, they are a lot like that sturdy tree. Winds blow, storms come, all kinds of hard things happen (maybe even a bird poops on it), but that tree stays solid

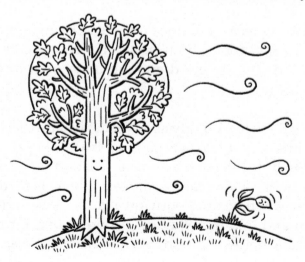

and strong. Kids who don't feel good inside often feel very hurt when something rough happens to them. They are **Wiggly as a Weed** in a storm.

When kids are **Strong as a Tree**, they still think they are okay when they get a less-than-perfect grade, or get in trouble, or get picked on—even though they might be unhappy about those things. But when kids who are **Wiggly as a Weed** get a less-than-perfect grade or get picked on, they think they are not okay. They feel bad, so they think they *are* bad. They blame themselves for everything that happens to them, even though hard things happen to everybody.

Imagine what it would feel like if you were **Strong as a Tree**. See if you can feel it right now. How would you stand if you felt strong inside? Imagine someone saying something unkind to you and see what it would feel like to be **Strong as a Tree**.

Being **Strong as a Tree** does not mean being a bully. It means feeling good about yourself, feeling confident, feeling like you are good enough and equal to everyone else.

Last year, Ryan felt **Wiggly as a Weed**. He didn't feel good about himself at all. When he got a bad grade at school, he tried to hide it from his mom and ended up getting in lots of trouble. This year, Ryan feels like he is **Strong as a Tree**, so when he did poorly on a quiz, he went right to his mom and told her. She was proud of him for telling her, and she helped him understand his mistakes.

When you are **Strong as a Tree**, you handle problems instead of hiding them, or you get help figuring out how to handle them. When you are **Wiggly as a Weed**, you hide your problems and feel bad about yourself.

Isabella got picked on at school. Some kids were really mean to her, and she felt terrible about herself and didn't want to go to school anymore. She felt like she was **Wiggly as a Weed** but she didn't want to feel that way. She wanted to become **Strong as a Tree**. So she told her mom how she felt. Isabella's mom decided to find a counselor Isabella could talk to. The counselor reminded Isabella that she was a good person and that those kids were being mean because they had their own problems and were trying to make themselves feel better by making someone else feel bad. With a lot of help from the counselor, she began to feel better about herself and focus on the kids who were nice to her. All of this helped Isabella to feel **Strong as a Tree**. When the mean kids approached her again, she thought to herself, *I don't deserve this*, and she got up, walked away, and found a friendlier kid to hang out with.

Most of the time would you say you feel **Strong as a Tree** *or* **Wiggly as a Weed**?

If you picked wiggly, how do you think it would feel inside to be **Strong as a Tree**?

Think of one thing you would do differently if you felt **Strong as a Tree**.

Spell Breaker #18:
Wild Horses, Buzzing Bees,
Flittering Flies, or Nasty Gnats

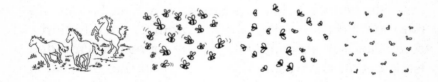

The Unkind Mind can be very powerful and feel really, really true. For some kids, the Unkind Mind can feel as powerful as **Wild Horses**, impossible to tame or quiet down. You might feel this, too. But over time, if you keep practicing all these Spell Breakers, you will find that your Unkind Mind has less and less power.

One sign that your Unkind Mind is getting less powerful is that it goes from feeling like **Wild Horses** to **Buzzing Bees**. **Buzzing Bees** can be painful and annoying but they aren't as strong as **Wild Horses**. And if you keep practicing these Spell Breakers, the unkind thoughts will become even weaker and less painful—more like **Flittering Flies** than **Buzzing Bees**. When this happens, your thoughts won't sting you like they did and you will have more time in your Kind Mind and Quiet Mind. Then, if you keep practicing even more, the Unkind Mind will only show up once in a while (maybe when life feels especially hard). Your unkind thoughts will become so small that they will feel more like tiny **Nasty Gnats** that you can just shoo away.

Then, if you keep going, someday you will be completely free of all these annoying pests and unkind thoughts. You will be free to just be a kid again: to play, hang out, go to school and simply be yourself.

These changes happen differently for everyone. Some kids find their minds moving pretty quickly from **Wild Horses** to **Buzzing Bees** to **Flittering Flies** to **Nasty Gnats**. For other kids, it takes longer. They may have been caught in the spell longer, so it might take more time for them to break it. Or they might have had more painful things happen in their lives, so the spell hangs on, trying to help them avoid their painful feelings. But everyone can become free.

On the path to becoming free, sometimes you might find yourself moving forward and sometimes you might find yourself standing still or even moving backwards. When this happens, it's important to remember that breaking the "I Feel Fat" Spell doesn't always happen easily…but that doesn't mean it's not happening. Two important words we teach kids to remember when they feel like they aren't getting better fast enough are "Not Yet!" So, the next time you feel like it is *never* going to get quiet in your mind, try telling yourself, *Not yet… but someday!*

Hailey started out feeling like her Unkind Mind had the power of **Wild Horses**. No matter what she tried, she could not quiet her Unkind Mind. "Not yet!" we reminded her. This helped her to not give up. And so she kept practicing Follow the Clues and Retrain Your Brain. She kept bringing herself back to what was Really Real and Sticking to the Facts. And then one day, Hailey came in and said, "It feels more like **Buzzing Bees** now!" After more practice with Slip 'n Slide and Just Say Yes, she said her Unkind Mind was starting to feel like **Flittering Flies**. When she started to get frustrated that she wasn't fully free, she would remind herself, *Not yet!* Over time, Hailey's Unkind Mind became weaker and weaker, which made it so much easier to ignore. At this point, she could easily shoo her unkind thoughts away, as if they were little **Nasty Gnats**. She was spending more and more time in freedom and what was Really Real and she continued to practice her favorite Spell Breakers. And then one day she came in and said, "I'm free! I don't think bad thoughts about my body anymore!" Now this doesn't mean Hailey will never again think an unkind thought, but when she does, she knows how to talk back to those thoughts and quiet them down again. She knows how it feels to be free and so can you!

Which of these best describes what your Unkind Mind feels like: **Wild Horses, Buzzing Bees, Flittering Flies, or Nasty Gnats**? *Or are you free of your Unkind Mind right now?*

Are you more free of the "I Feel Fat" Spell than when you started reading this book?

When do you feel most free from the spell?

Spell Breaker #19: How Would I Be If I Were Free?

Sometimes it takes a while to break the "I Feel Fat" Spell. So, until it is broken, and you are free again, you can use your imagination to try on your new way of being. In Spell Breaker #10, you learned about Mind Movies and how to Change the Channel when your mind is playing a painful movie. In this Spell Breaker, you will learn to play *positive* Mind Movies that will help you practice feeling better until you *are* better.

When someone is going to build a house they picture what they want in their mind. This helps them figure out how to build it. When you imagine how it would be if you were free of the spell, you will start to move in that direction. This Spell Breaker teaches you the power of your imagination when you ask yourself, ***How Would I Be If I Were Free?***

For example, if you have a hard time deciding what to wear to school in the morning, you can ask yourself, ***How Would I Be If I Were Free?*** What would be different? How would you feel? What would it be like to get dressed if you were free of the spell?

Or, if you feel really uncomfortable in your body, try imagining how it would be if you felt really good and comfortable in your body. Using your imagination to practice how it feels to be free will help you actually *become* free.

Caitlin told us she knew she was under the spell when she got dressed in the morning. Her Unkind Mind told her over and over that she was too fat and looked terrible. This made it very hard for her to get dressed. Sometimes, it even made her late for school. So Caitlin tried this Spell Breaker and asked herself, **How Would I Be If I Were Free?** She said she would just look in her closet and pick out something that she felt like wearing that day. Maybe she'd choose a color she was in the mood for or, depending on the weather, something cooler or warmer. Caitlin said that if she were free, she wouldn't stress about how she looked; she would focus on being comfortable. It would be easy and fun to get dressed. All her clothes would be equal because she would know that she is good enough just as she is. So, she tried on this new way of thinking, just like she tried on her school clothes in the morning. Eventually, the new way replaced the old way, and she no longer had a hard time getting dressed for the day!

Lily noticed that she was in her Unkind Mind when she was comparing herself to other kids at school and thinking she was bigger or uglier. She asked herself, **How Would I Be If I Were Free?** Her answer was, "If I were free, I would remember that it's Unfair to Compare and I would stop comparing myself to others. I would feel fine just the way I am!" It took Lily a little while before this new way of thinking became real but trying it on in her mind helped her to get there.

Luke sometimes ate too much. Ashley was afraid to eat. Both kids asked themselves, *How Would I Be If I Were Free?* and they both came up with the same answer: "I would listen to my body and eat when I'm hungry and stop when I'm full!" Thinking about this helped both Luke and Ashley to start listening more to their bodies and eating the amount of food their bodies really needed.

Josh was making himself exercise too much because he thought if he changed his body he would look better and have more friends. So, when Josh asked himself, *How Would I Be If I Were Free?* he realized he would exercise a normal amount, only in gym class and while playing with friends, and he wouldn't worry about it all the time. After a while, Josh began exercising the way he imagined, just for fitness and fun, and he stopped worrying about it. As Josh broke free of the "I Feel Fat" Spell, all the peace he had imagined started to come true.

How would you be if you were free?

What are some things you do that make you think you are under the "I Feel Fat" Spell?

*Pick one of those things and ask yourself, **How Would I Be If I Were Free?***

Now, spend some time imagining what that would really feel and be like.

Spell Breaker #20:
Be a Body Buddy

If you have been caught by the "I Feel Fat" Spell, you might focus so much on what you don't like about your body that you forget about all the good things your body does for you.

Did you know...

Your heart beats around 100,000 times a day?

There are around 650 skeletal muscles in the human body?

It takes 17 muscles in the face for us to smile (and 43 muscles to frown)?[1]

Our bodies are really cool and super busy. They are working for us all the time so that we can enjoy our lives and get things done. So, don't you think it's a little bit strange for us to be mean to our bodies when they work so hard for us?

---

[1] "Muscle Facts for Kids." *Science Kids*. 2015.

Imagine telling your best friend, "You're so fat. You're gross. Your stomach sticks out." They probably wouldn't want to be your friend anymore! So how friendly do you think it is to let your Unkind Mind pick on your body and make you feel bad all the time?

What if you could become a better friend to your body? What if you could learn how to talk to your body like you talk to your best buddy? What if you could become a **Body Buddy**?

Even if you have trouble liking parts of your body right now, you can still find other things about it that you like. Your body helps you play and get around. It has five amazing senses that help you hear, touch, taste, smell, and see all the beautiful and special things around you.

When you start saying nice things about your body, it makes your mind more peaceful. When you start saying nice things *and* stop saying mean things to your body, you become a **Body Buddy**. Kids who are **Body Buddies** are super cool. They are happier than people who aren't **Body Buddies,** and they are better able to resist the "I Feel Fat" Spell.

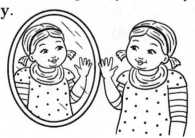

Here are some things that **Body Buddies** do:

Smile when they look in the mirror.

Focus on the parts of their bodies they like and not on the parts they don't like.

Stop themselves when they notice they are thinking mean things about their bodies.

Appreciate their bodies for all the amazing things they do.

Remind themselves that they are lovable no matter how they look today.

Do nice things for their bodies: get enough sleep, have enough (but not too much) physical activity, rest when tired.

Eat when they are hungry, stop eating when they start to feel full.

Eat fruits, vegetables, proteins, carbohydrates and fats.

No matter what size or shape your body is, it deserves a **Body Buddy!**

Think of something you did today that made you happy. How did your body help you do it?

What are three things you like about your body?

Now close your eyes and tell your body one of those things.

See how easy it is to become a **Body Buddy?**

Spell Breaker #21:
Mirror, Mirror on the Wall

Well, you have almost made it to the end of this book. Good job! Hopefully, you have learned many different ways to stand up to your **Unkind Mind** and are spending more time in your **Quiet Mind**. Hopefully you are remembering that **It's Unfair to Compare,** and you are becoming a **Body Buddy.** You are the only one in the world who is just like you, and you have only one body to live in. So, can you **Just Say Yes** to it?

We hope you are spending more time in what is **Really Real** and less time in **Mind Movies.** And hopefully you are remembering to **Follow the Clues** when the "I Feel Fat" Spell strikes you. Are you able to catch **Fat Chat** when you or others are doing it? And when someone hurts your feelings, are you able to **Slip 'n Slide** or **Say What You Mean but Don't Say It Mean?** Remember, **Stick to the Facts** so you don't get lost in your feelings, and don't forget that **Fat is Not a Feeling!**

We hope you have broken free of the "I Feel Fat" Spell, but if not, we hope it's feeling more like **Buzzing Bees, Flittering Flies, or Nasty Gnats.** If you can't feel love for your body yet, that's okay. You can try again tomorrow… and the next day after that! You can keep practicing until you get good at it. Just remember that, like anything, you have to practice to get better. So keep practicing all these **Spell Breakers** and get help with the ones that are super hard for you. You *can* break free of the "I Feel Fat" Spell!

*What are your three favorite **Spell Breakers**?*

What is one thing that has changed for you since you started practicing these Spell Breakers?

What is the most important thing you've learned from reading this book?

Spell Breaker #22: Wellness Wizards

If you are feeling free, or at least freer than when you started this book, we hope you will give yourself lots of credit. But, if you are still caught in the "I Feel Fat" Spell, we'd like you to think about finding what we call a **"Wellness Wizard."**

A **Wellness Wizard** is someone who can help you break free of your Unkind Mind. When you have a hurt tooth, you go to the dentist. When you are sick, you go to the doctor. When grown-ups have car problems, they take their cars to the mechanic. Well, when kids are not thinking good thoughts about their precious bodies, they need a **Wellness Wizard.**

A **Wellness Wizard** is someone you feel safe and comfortable with, someone you can talk to about your most difficult thoughts and feelings. That might be one or both of your parents. It could be a counselor at school or somewhere else. It might even be a favorite relative you really trust. There are lots of people who can help you—you just have to find them, or have somebody help you find them, and use your courage to tell them the truth about how you are feeling.

Who do you feel safe talking to about your feelings?

Would you like your parents to find you someone really wise and kind you can talk to?

We are so glad you took the time to read this book. We hope you will read it again and again so that you can learn lots of **Spell Breakers** and live peacefully ever after (and know what to do when you aren't!).

One Final Note

Caitlin's "I Feel Fat" Spell used to be as strong as **Wild Horses**. When she was caught in the spell, she would look in the mirror and say the meanest things to herself, but not anymore. After learning and practicing all of the **Spell Breakers**, she now feels free. These days, she looks in the mirror and sings this little song:

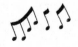

Mirror, Mirror on the wall
I can get up if I fall

My body is a wonderful thing
I can laugh or cry or dance or sing

The Mirror Witch was very wrong
My body and I now get along

We all have muscles, bones, and fat
All bodies are beautiful and that is that

It's not about the way I look
I changed my thinking, that's what it took

Life is better when I say yes to me
Life is better 'cuz now I'm free

Note to Parents

It used to be that mainly adults got struck by the "I Feel Fat" Spell, but now children far and wide are getting caught in its grips. While many books and theories cast blame on parents for much of what happens to their child, it is entirely possible that your kid's body image problem has more to do with our crazy culture and *their* individual personality than with your parenting or your personality.

If your child is emotionally sensitive, achievement-oriented, and has a people-pleasing personality, they may be especially susceptible to the "I Feel Fat" Spell. Children with these tendencies want to do their best, and if they think that means weight loss, toned thighs, and flat abs, well, they're on it. If, on top of being a sensitive kid with a need to please, your child has had painful experiences they don't know how to navigate and communicate, there's a likelihood they could develop body obsession as a distraction from these deeper issues. So, despite what you may have been told, it's entirely possible that your child's problem has little or nothing to do with you.

On the other hand, it's possible that you may be innocently contributing to your child's body image problem. Given our cultural obsession with thinness and accompanying fat phobia, there's a good chance that you, too, may be struggling with body image. If you diet, binge, eat emotionally, dislike your body, or judge other people based on their looks, you may be teaching these things to your child. If you are making negative comments about your own body, your child, who may not be fully emotionally separated from you, may think something is wrong with her body. If you are using food, or food restriction, to calm your own anxiety, your child will not be learning healthy ways to calm his.

Another way that parents can unwittingly contribute to a child's body image problem is by discouraging them from expressing their emotions. While it's important to teach kids to control themselves, they also need to learn how to express what needs to be expressed. Otherwise, they may use food, food restriction, or body obsession to numb or distract from their emotions.

It is critical that we adults be how we want our children to be. So if you want your child to love her body, you will need to work on loving yours. If you want your child to eat normally, work on doing that yourself. If you want your child to value movement and activity, make sure you are not over—or under—doing it. If you want your child to be healthy in his expression of emotions, make sure you get your own support to do the same.

We hope this book will help your child break free from the "I Feel Fat" Spell, and we hope we have inspired you with new ways to help your child. May you both learn to love the bodies you live in. May we all live healthily ever after.

Parental Potions:
How to Reverse the Curse in Your Home

Demonstrate a non-diet, moderate, enjoyable relationship with food.

Practice listening to your body's needs for both movement and rest.

Get help for yourself if you recognize that you, too, have issues with food, weight, or body image that you can't resolve on your own.

If your child is overeating or undereating, educate yourself on how to help children with their emotions, as well as how to teach kids *Intuitive Eating*. There are many books, blogs, counselors, and (non-diet) dieticians that can help.

When teaching your child about nutrition, keep a positive approach. Fear and shame-based approaches tend to backfire.

Make sure to address unresolved family pain through counseling, spiritual advice, or education so that your child doesn't use food or weight to act out family issues.

Refrain from talking about dieting and weight loss. Talking about these topics increases the likelihood that your child will develop disordered eating.

Focus on enjoying a wide variety of foods, in moderation, and creating a non-judgmental atmosphere around eating.

Let friends and relatives know that your child is sensitive to messages about food and weight, and request that they abstain from weight comments and diet-talk (Fat Chat) in front of your kid.

Refrain from verbalizing anything negative about your body or other peoples' bodies in hearing-distance of your kid. (Or, better yet, at all!) Expressing a positive, grateful attitude about your body will increase the chances that your child will do the same.

Learn how to become a good listener so when your child comes to you with difficult emotions, you can respond in the most helpful ways.

About the Authors

Andrea's Story:

Children are not born with a bad body image. They learn it. They learn it from the culture and the media, or from relatives, friends, and schoolmates who learned it from the culture and the media. And since body hatred is an epidemic in our image-obsessed culture, there is no shortage of places for kids to learn to dislike their bodies. As a psychotherapist who has been specializing in eating disorders for over 25 years, I have been helping people of all ages who battle with their bodies to varying degrees. Whether they are dealing with a full-blown eating disorder, less severe "disordered eating," or painful body image issues, they all deserve and need help.

I began hating my body when I was twelve years old. Someone teased me about the size of my thighs, and I felt what I now know was shame for the first time. This is what I refer to as a "Dart in the Heart" moment. My solution was to embark on my very first diet. Like many, this led me to sneak eating, bingeing, and roller coaster weight fluctuations. Like some, this morphed into a serious eating disorder. I say serious because it colored most of my life for several decades and greatly affected my mental and physical well-being. Fortunately, after many years of searching for help that actually helped, I began to unravel the root causes of my eating disorder and body obsession. I learned that I could not stop bingeing if I did not stop dieting. I learned what emotions I was eating over and what to do with those emotions instead. I learned how to challenge rather than believe every thought that popped up on the screen of my mind. And I learned how to find sweetness from many different sources, not just from cookies and ice cream. It was a long road. And the lovely parting gift from that arduous journey is that I now have the honor of helping others who struggle in similar ways.

The majority of my clients over the last few decades have been teenagers, college students, and adults, with a small sprinkling of young kids. But as our cultural obsessions with thinness, dieting, fat phobia, and social media have all gotten bigger, the age range of my clients seems to be getting younger. So instead of getting occasional calls from concerned parents, counselors, and doctors, I now receive them regularly. Imagine a small six-year-old child who cannot get dressed for school in the morning because she thinks she's too "fat," or an eleven-year-old girl who won't go to a sleepover because all her friends are thinner than she is. Imagine a lovely eight-year-old who once enjoyed swimming but will no longer go in the pool because she feels too self-conscious in a bathing suit, or a nine-year-old boy who, though underweight, refuses to eat carbs. Or how about an eight-year-old girl who is obsessed with working out?

When I was eight years old, I was blissfully unaware of my body. I was playing tag in the yard with my siblings or watching The Brady Bunch in the den. I listened to records. I read in my canopy bed. Today, many young kids are surfing the Internet on iPhones and computers. This means that on top of the brainwashing they get on television, they are ingesting an additional barrage of messages on their other screens. They are bombarded with information about unnatural thinness, fat phobia, excessive fitness, endless food rules, and adult sexuality. Most of us adults did not experience anything like this until we were much older. And even then, we found it difficult to get through unscathed.

As I began to see more young children each week, I found myself needing to adapt the work I had been doing with adults into a more "kid-friendly" version. Some of the parents reported that they had already taken the advice from the current self-help literature: limiting screen time, filtering media, and teaching their children that all bodies are beautiful. While these suggestions are great, they weren't helping to change what was already going on with their kids. It was as if their children had fallen under a spell, and nothing these parents said seemed to make any difference. What we needed to do was find a way to break the spell, or Retrain the Brain.

So, as I began teaching kids how to talk back to their Unkind Minds and strengthen their Kind Minds, I began to see something really exciting. Week after week, these precious little munchkins were bouncing into my office exclaiming that what we were doing was making a difference! One little six-year-old literally skipped into my office and said, "I was totally free this week. I think we broke the spell. It feels so much better to be in reality!" Another child, when I asked her to describe to her mom what she was learning in our sessions said, "Well, I was under the spell 98% last week, and this week I'm only 73% spell." (Sounds like a budding mathematician to me!) One young boy, during a family session, announced, "I am over it. I'm sick of being so hard on myself. I just want to eat normally from now on. I don't want to have to be perfect." One parent told me that his daughter, who had been refusing to wear sleeveless dresses and bathing suits, was swimming again and taking off the oversized jackets that had become her daily cover-ups.

All of these dramatic changes were confirmation to me that there is great hope for children with painful body images. I realized I simply had to write a book to share these ideas and exercises with other children, parents, and counselors. It has been an honor to share with you all the tips and tools that helped me break my own spell, and I sincerely hope that this book will help the child you care about break free of theirs.

Marsea's Story:

My tortured relationship with my body began when I was thirteen. I used to think that was very young, but I now recognize that had I grown up in today's world, it would have probably hit me at a much younger age. It seemed to me at the time (though I realize in hindsight, inaccurately) that I was bigger than the other girls around me, and I assumed this meant I was "fat" and I further assumed that it was very bad to be fat. I didn't know then that I was just naturally softer and fleshier than some of my girlfriends, much like my wonderful grandma. But in 1972, hot pants, hip huggers, mini-skirts, and tube tops were the fashion, and Twiggy had recently retired at the top of her game. I didn't understand that, even at my healthiest possible weight, I would never look like Twiggy nor would I ever look good in a tube top (and that these things were perfectly okay). What I did understand was that all the women in my family were dieting, and it seemed reasonable that if I were to fit properly in the world around me, I would need to diet as well. So I embarked on a dieting career that would last for almost two decades. And I was pretty good at it, following each and every instruction and rule to the bitter end. Unfortunately, I had the bad "luck" of being one of the 98% of people who, after the successful completion of a diet, re-gain all their lost weight, plus a little more. Not realizing it was *dieting* that was the problem, I mistakenly thought I was a miserable failure.

Looking back, I realize that my *original* problem had little to do with weight and nothing to do with eating. My actual problem had four parts to it. First, due to heredity and genetics, my body was never meant to be anything like the tiny girls around me. My body was and will always be the fleshy type, with large breasts and a bit of a "Buddha belly"—more of an "oak tree" than a "redwood." My second problem was that I was insecure. I didn't understand that I was lovable and attractive, regardless of my size. I thought that my flabby belly was an obstacle to love and success. I felt ashamed, anxious, and completely unacceptable as a person. I didn't have a secure sense of my "okay-ness." The third part of the problem was that I didn't know how to deal with or communicate these painful feelings. I'm sure I looked like I was a happy, healthy person. I did my best to pretend that I was. I hid my anxiety and shame. In fact, though I didn't know it, I was stuffing these feelings down with food. But even more important than that was problem number four—I didn't know how to connect with people, have intimate relationships, and share my authentic feelings. I thought that life was about how I looked, not about how I connected with myself and others.

Because I dieted to keep my weight down, no one knew that I had an eating disorder. In fact, I got nothing but praise for all the exercising and dieting that I did. People admired me for being so strong and disciplined and even asked me for tips on how they could lose weight like I did. In other words, I actually got support for being on the wrong track! It took getting to the point of uncontrollable daily binges, a 75-lb. weight gain, and severe depression for me to realize that I needed, and could get, help. And I finally understood that "help" wasn't another diet, it was psychological help. I basically had to learn that everything I thought about eating, dieting and weight had been misguided. I had essentially been brainwashed by the dieting industry and all my efforts to be a good dieter had led to nothing but misery and weight gain. I had to completely Retrain My Brain and break the spell that dieting had on me. I took this journey when I was in my late twenties.

Many years later, when I became a therapist, I found it fairly easy to work with people in their twenties and older. But as more parents began calling for help with their young children, I found myself stymied about how to help them. I didn't know how to put the adult concepts of eating disorder recovery into words that kids could relate to. So when Andrea started using Fairy Tales, child-friendly language, and rhyming phrases that her young clients were absorbing and utilizing, I knew she was onto something. And given my own need for resources in helping kids, I jumped excitedly into this project.

Today, as a culture, we are much more aware of eating disorders. We know that a person actually *can* be too thin. (Remember the phrase "You can never be too rich or too thin?") We no longer glamorize anorexia in quite the way we used to. We recognize that young children should not be obsessed with their weight. But, unfortunately, more and more are. This book is our attempt to speak to children in their own language, to help them make a distinction between their true selves and their Unkind Minds, and to inspire them to stand up to our cultural obsession with weight and perfectionism.

Acknowledgments

Andrea would like to thank:

My dear family and friends who have supported my work and my writing since day one. You loved and believed in me when I was deeply caught in the spell, and I am forever grateful.

My extraordinary business partner, Marsea Marcus. I could not have asked for someone with more integrity, wisdom, and skill. Thank you for taking this journey with me.

Julia V. Taylor for igniting the spark that inspired me to create this book and for generously allowing us to use her *Hurtful Comparisons* exercise.

My precious mom and my amazing sister, Lori Wachter Wolfson, for reading the manuscript and giving us your valuable feedback.

My sister-in-law, Katie Hafner for leading me to Booktrope. Your editing, cheerleading, and literary leads have been invaluable.

All the devoted and gifted teachers who have helped me retrain my own brain and break free from the spell: Eckhart Tolle, Leonard Jacobson, Byron Katie, Esther Hicks, and Lester Levenson.

My wonderful husband, Steve Legallet, for your constant encouragement, support, love, and levity. I am so lucky I get to live my life with you.

All the parents who have trusted me with their precious kids. It is because of you and your children's willingness to go see "some lady" that the ideas in this book became tried and true. It really does take a village, and I am honored to be part of yours.

Marsea would like to thank:

First and foremost, Evan Rotman, for loving me, supporting me in all it took to complete this book, and making me laugh every. single. day.

My mother for her endless love, support, and generosity.

My father for his unceasing kindness and positive attitude, and for teaching me "Moderation in all things, including moderation!"

Erica Golden for her inspiration and editing advice. There is nothing like an old friend who transcends time and space.

My individual and group clients who honor me with their vulnerability and their trust. I am so fortunate to know each and every one of you, and I delight in your growth and healing.

And, finally, to Andrea Wachter, my undying gratitude for your organized nature, amazing ability to keep us moving forward on all projects big and small, and your boundless enthusiasm and positive outlook. I am deeply honored that you invited me to join you on yet another exciting journey.

Andrea and Marsea would both like to thank:

Francie White, an extraordinary healer who has pioneered the way for so much of the work that we do. Francie is the author of the original Mirror Witch Tale, and as a Storyteller herself, she welcomed our adaptation of her story. Francie, your feedback on the manuscript was priceless. You are a gem.

Carolyn Costin, another gifted pioneer in the eating disorder field. Thank you for all the work you have done, the books you have published, and for your helpful insights about our cover.

Jenni McGuire for your generous editorial assistance.

My sister-in-law, Katie Hafner, for your invaluable editing, cheerleading, and literary leads.

Our wonderful team at Booktrope for helping this book come to fruition:

Heather Huffman, your kindness, promptness, professionalism, and big heart have been such a gift.

Amanda Gawthorpe, your quick wit, your way with words, and your knowledge of grammar are all extremely appreciated.

Tim Derrig, we so appreciate you joining our team mid-stream and helping us get this book out to those in need of it.

Emerald Barnes for believing in the importance of this topic and fitting us into your very full schedule.

Michelle Fairbanks, your artistic talent has been a perfect match for us. We are so grateful to have found you.

And thank you to Jennifer Kalis for your wonderfully playful, light-hearted, yet meaningful illustrations.

Author Bios

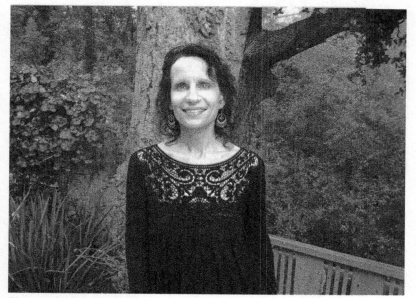

Photo credit: Steve Legallet

Andrea Wachter, LMFT is a licensed psychotherapist who specializes in eating disorders, depression, anxiety, and grief. Andrea is the author of *Getting Over Overeating for Teens* and is a regular contributor to *The Huffington Post*. Andrea is an inspirational counselor, author, and speaker who uses professional expertise, humor, and personal recovery to help others. For more information on her books, blogs, or other services, please visit: www.andreawachter.com.

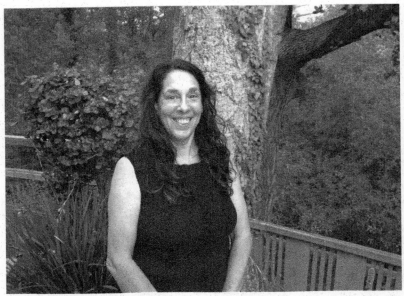

Photo credit: Steve Legallet

Marsea Marcus, LMFT is a licensed therapist and author specializing in the healing of eating disorders, sexual abuse, trauma, and depression. She obtained her Master's degree from John F. Kennedy University. She is a trained Process Therapist and is also certified in the use of EMDR, a trauma therapy. Marsea has worked in several inpatient treatment centers for eating disorders and addiction recovery. She also maintains a private practice in Northern California.

Both authors are co-founders of InnerSolutions Counseling Services and co-authors of *The Don't Diet, Live-It! Workbook*. To learn more, go to: www.innersolutions.net.

CPSIA information can be obtained
at www.ICGtesting.com
Printed in the USA
LVOW03s1611071117
555372LV00002B/388/P